HOW TO TAKE A CRISIS AND BUILD A SOLID *Foundation*

PERSONAL THEORETICAL FRAMEWORK FOR *Application in Practice*

SHELLY LYNN PETERS

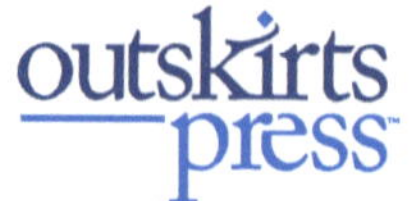

TABLE OF CONTENTS

INTRODUCTION

PSYCHOTHERAPY PROVES TO assist human beings to care for themselves and others methodically; and articulations of these theories have been studied and utilized for decades to offer effective treatment to troubled individuals. This essay presents three theories favored to implement in a professional practice. Carl Rogers, Aaron Beck, and Marsha Linehan are discussed for their qualities of therapy from original conception, major concepts, and diagrams that reflect their methods of psychotherapy.

Components of each theory that are most appealing have been identified and implemented into a personal theoretical framework. The step-by-step concepts are developed into a diagram for a visual overall understanding that will be applied to a diverse population of mental health seeking clients. A brief case is introduced as an example of a client situation where this method will be exercised to reveal the process of personal regard, growth and development, and actualization. Lastly, a simple critique including strengths, limitations, and utilization of the therapeutic process identified is discussed.

ORIGIN OF THEORIES

PERSON-CENTERED THERAPY (PCT) was pioneered by Carl Rogers in the 1940s from the culminating events of his personal experiences. His feelings related to a rigid upbringing in a fundamentalist Protestantism combined with his seminarian experience led him to stand his ground with developing genuine caring relationships with clients. Rogers was preparing for a profession as clergy, after a couple of years studying religion and theology he transitioned into the field of psychology and in 1931 received his PhD. Rogers was inspired through the work of Otto Rank (1936) whose view was the therapist ought to be humane in working with the problems of people more so than exercising their technical skills. Research was conducted in the 1950s-1960s leading to the recognition of therapists' genuine self-disclosure as an effective method leading to more positive outcomes for the clients. (Prochaska, 2014) Rogers was a peace-maker highly involved with "humanistic changes in education, business, marriage, and world relations". He believed that "clients (not 'patients') are the ones who possess the resources for change; adopting a nondirective, egalitarian approach to promote personal growth within the individuals seeking therapy". Rogers was well known for "validating a person's sense of worth" (Farber, 1996).

Dialectical behavior therapy (DBT) originated with Marsha Linehan in the 1970s conceived through reflection of her personal experience as an inpatient in a long-term residential treatment program related to personal infliction of injury at age 17 "for what would now likely be diagnosed as Borderline Personality Disorder (BPD)". Linehan purposed to treat clients diagnosed with BPD and so pursued a PhD in experimental personality psychology at Loyola University in 1971 (Prochaska, 2014). As with Rogers, Linehan's therapy is supported by research as the main treatment effective in decreasing suicidal behavior, and is the "gold-standard treatment for BPD of which has an 8-10 suicide rate" (Facuty of Department of Psychology, 2011). Linehan too, has a foundation of faith that supports her passion to grow in the understanding of humanity. Linehan lived, learned, and exposed the concept of "radical acceptance", coming to terms with who she is. She reveals to the New York Times (2011) her personal experience living with a mental disorder overcoming the fear of speaking the truth about her own past diagnosis and sharing her path of recovery. This path of personal growth and development became the catalyst for the development of DBT. Linehan knows firsthand the "discipline of behaviorism taught that people could learn new behaviors — and that acting differently can in time alter underlying emotions from the top down" (Carey, 2011).

Cognitive behavioral therapy (CBT) finds its origination in the 1960s with psychologist Aaron Beck who "discovered that by teaching patients to examine and test their negative ideas, their depression began to improve". Like Rogers and Linehan, Beck was involved in research although that of psychoanalysis to formulate a "cognitive theory and therapy for mental disorders". Beck was focused on guiding clients to become aware of their maladaptive perceptions. Beck associated "maladaptive cognitions, dysfunctional attitudes, or depressogenic assumptions" as the leading role in several mental disorders. Beck also has personal experience with trauma as a young boy thus leading to "fears of abandonment and health-related phobias". Beck went on to test his cognitive theory by exposing himself to fearful situations. (Prochaska, 2014) Beck's creative system of psychotherapy continues to be promoted and supported through research and his daughter, Dr. Judith Beck, president of the Beck Institute of Cognitive Therapy provides professional education and training in CBT.

Major Concepts and Components

ROGERS'S PERSON-CENTERED therapy stands up under the umbrella of the theory of personality. Actualization, Rogers believes, unlike Freud, that humans have an established pattern of behavior to exercise growth, to develop through "relating and reproducing". Key is the ability to transition from external controlling forces into internal controls. Rogers believed we are born with organismic valuing, the ability to perceive the positive and negative experiences that motivates us; and we can trust these intrinsic motivations. Coming to terms with our self-consciousness and learning self-regard. Rogers' goal was to establish the sense of worth to the individual. He posits humans learn to trade actualization for conditional love; this being the seed of psychopathology. Of utmost importance is the therapeutic relationship. There are six principles required for the foundation of this relationship that support the therapeutic personality change:

1. Relationship involving reciprocity.
2. Vulnerability to anxiety causes the person to maintain the therapeutic relationship.
3. Genuineness of the therapist includes self-expression.
4. Unconditional positive regard, leading the person to develop awareness of previously distortion or denied regard from significant others.
5. Accurate empathy allows us to sense the others personal world as though it were our own without the fear, anger, and confusion surrounding us.
6. Perception of genuineness by the person with acceptance and understanding of the therapist. (Prochaska, 2014)

Rogers's therapeutic processes involve consciousness raising and catharsis. Within the relationship the client is free to discuss anything during the session and thus direct the flow of therapy; labeled nondirective. The therapist has the responsibility of raising the client's awareness through reflection. The attention given to the client's feelings aids the client to "break through their perceptual distortions in order to attend to the personal meaning of experiences that previously have not been processed into awareness" (Prochaska, 2014). Catharsis involves helping the person own their feelings and allowing them expression and "release of the emotional component of feelings" (Prochaska, 2014).

Linehan's dialectical behavior therapy is developed with the cornerstone of Rogers's person-centered therapy; she realized the principles of behavior change must be balanced with genuine regard. Major concepts include mindfulness and meditation. Consciousness raising, choosing, and counterconditioning make up the general steps involved in the therapeutic process. Consciousness raising according to Linehan affords the client the learning opportunity to observe and discern their personal environment, be it internal or external. This discernment must be practiced as non-judgmental so the client can describe their observation and assist others with awareness. Clients then learn to participate in the now and not focusing on the past distressing events. Choosing encompasses the fact that all humans will experience pain, loneliness, frustration, disease, and death at some point in their lives; choosing to accept it verses avoidance is processed with mindfulness. Acceptance of who we are is chosen over the continuous dread of the past and future perceived circumstances. DBT teaches several different skill sets to accompany the therapeutic process including emotional regulation, interpersonal effectiveness, and radical acceptance. DBTs therapeutic relationship includes validation strategies like Rogers and the dialectic may resemble balance with "warm and empathic and at times powerful and confrontational" (Prochaska, 2014). The progression of DBT therapy graduates from like parenting to teaching, then consulting.

Beck's cognitive behavior therapy is driven by the belief that psychopathology originates in the preconscious state; events are perceived through "cognitive lenses" that lead to mental distress. Beck recognized cognitive errors lead to depressing feelings; identified as depressogenic assumptions

- Overgeneralizing: if it's true in one situation, it applies to any situation remotely similar.
- Selective abstraction: the only events that matter are the failures, which are the sole measure of myself.
- Excessive responsibility: I am responsibility for all bad things, rotten events and life failures.
- Self-references: I am at the center of everyone's attention, particularly when I fail at something.

- Dichotomous thinking: everything is either one extreme or another (black or white, good or bad). (Prochaska, 2014)

CBT therapeutic relationship exercises the Socratic dialogue; clients are guided with questions in hopes of personal discovery. In this time of exploration, the individual find thoughts that are not accurate. CBT therapist's main role is the expert and director of treatment and client is the collaborator with responsibility for producing the treatments positive outcome. The client becomes the expert as principle applications are practiced. (Prochaska, 2014)

DIAGRAMS

PERSON-CENTERED THERAPY begins with genuine care for the client intending to assist them with recognizing that which is a dominant thought from external conditional love.

Carl Rogers's theory of actualization is primarily the process of becoming oneself – I am love from within.

Rogers posits humans learn to trade actualization for conditional love; thus leading to psychopathology.

Healing/recovery begins in the presence of one who practices positive regard, leading the person into awareness of distorted thoughts and denied regard from significant others.

Rogers's Person Centered Therapy Model

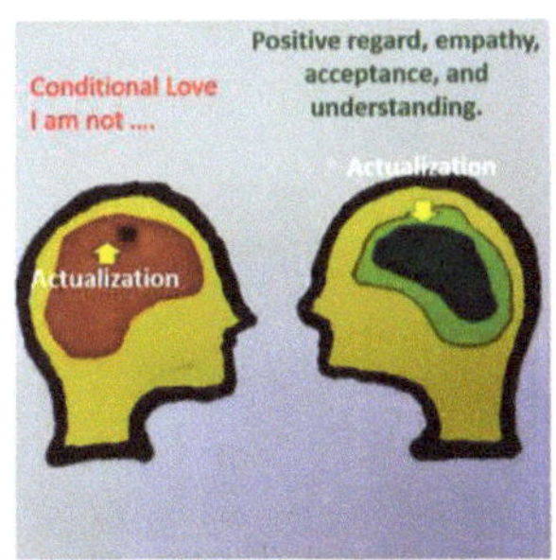

Figure 1 Positive regard, empathy, acceptance, and understanding.

Person-centered therapy begins with genuine care for the client intending to assist them with recognizing that which is a dominant thought from external conditional love.

Carl Rogers's theory of actualization is primarily the process of becoming oneself – I am love from within.

Rogers posits humans learn to trade actualization for conditional love; thus leading to psychopathology.

Healing/recovery begins in the presence of one who practices positive regard, leading the person into awareness of distorted thoughts and denied regard from significant others.

Linehan's Dialectical Behavior Therapy Model

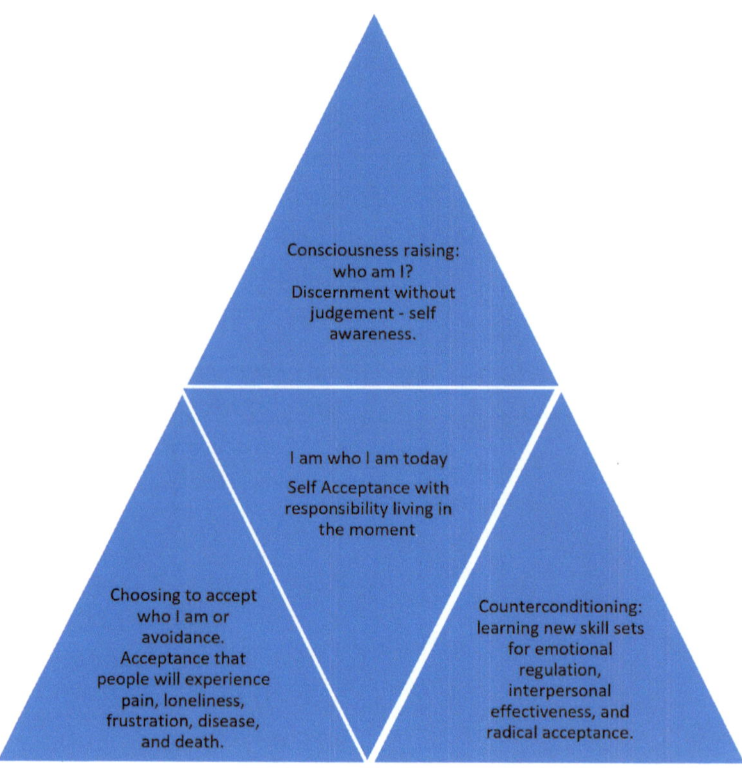

Principles of behavior change must be balanced with genuine regard from the therapist; the progression of therapeutic relationship is on toward consulting.

Beck's Cognitive Behavior Therapy Model

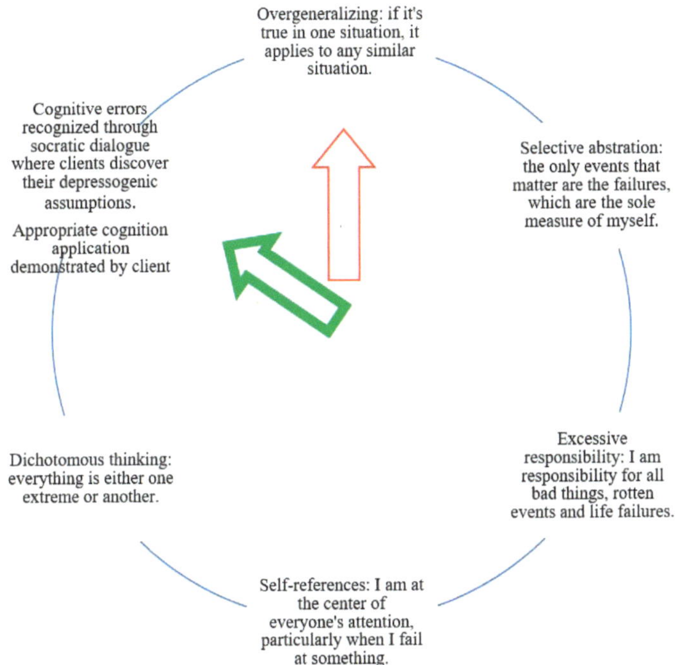

Learning how to think about what you are thinking summarizes CBT.

Chosen Components

THE THEORIES OF Rogers, Linehan, and Beck are chosen with the image of building a home and setting the foundation for a strong functional structure. Conscious raising and catharsis are seemingly common in the field of psychology and for good cause; they facilitate excavation of hard ground and are mined for recycled use. Continuing with the metaphor of construction, the relationship with the contractor is like the therapist and therapeutic relationship. Without the collaboration and wisdom of the therapist and client there is no mortar to bind the foundation.

Rogers's theory of the therapeutic relationship is a critical component to positive outcomes across the board of psychopathology. Indeed the intent of PCT is for a personality change although I would go as far as equating this to Linehan's radical self acceptance. It's not always a change in self that takes place but the invitation of meeting who you are and getting to know who you are; the process of personal growth and development. Here is where Beck's personal discovery through cognitive behavior therapy enters the scene.

Principles of CBT that will be utilized with my clients include:

- Based on an ever-evolving formulation of individual problems; considering client's current thinking, problematic behaviors and precipitating factors.
- Collaboration and active participation: includes willingness and ability to perform therapy homework outside of scheduled sessions.
- Goal oriented with problem focused measurable pathways.
- Emphasize the present- time problems.
- Educate the client to become one's own therapist; preventing relapse.
- Therapy sessions are timed and structured: introductory part, middle part, final part.
- Teach client to identify, evaluate, and respond appropriately to their dysfunctional thoughts and beliefs.

- CBT uses a variety of techniques to change thinking, mood, and behavior: homework is based on diagnosis. (Beck, 2011)

Beck and Linehan both offer education as a major concept leading to positive personal growth and development. Linehan however, is more complex and in depth with the intrinsic aspects of development not necessarily changing the person but teaching the individual to accept a reality that often involves a mental illness diagnosis.

Dialectical Behavior Therapy principles fittingly braid themselves with CBT, including four main skill sets:

- Mindfulness skills - teach how to observe and experience reality; these are the base of the DBT skill sets.
- Interpersonal Effectiveness skills - help manage interpersonal conflicts and maintain and improve relationships with others. Goal setting and identification of interference are examined and include obtaining objectives skillfully. Relationship building and ending destructive ones are covered as well as 'walking the middle path'.
- Emotion Regulation skills – helps to manage

emotions using tools that aid in understanding and naming emotions, changing emotional responses, reducing vulnerability to emotion mind, and managing really difficult emotions.
- Distress Tolerance skills – help to learn to tolerate and survive crisis situations without making things worse. (Lineham, 2015)

Linehan offers handouts and worksheets specific for each category to facility the process.

The rationale for choosing person-centered therapy, cognitive behavior therapy, and dialectical behavior therapy is how well they collaboratively enhance personal growth and development without regard for the individual's past. The goals of PCT, CBT, and DBT are to assist the individual to be in relationship with themselves; accepting and loving the 'I am'. Often people believe that because of past experience (regretful ones usually) they are unable to go forward and become all that is possible. Personal experience has taught me to accept all that I am. Metaphorically, like the Bible, it is not complete without the Old and New Testaments. It is not viewed for only good outcomes and clean-cut behaviors, but it is whole and accepted- 'the good, the bad, and the ugly'. Each of the therapies does not judge the individuals and teaches them self discipline and self regard.

The foundation diagram is designed to exhort a client to work from the basement up; as rushing ahead (or skipping steps) will likely lead to an unsteady self. Notice, as indicated in the essay that positive regard for self and worthy of love are pictured as the cornerstone. Without this critical element the other blocks will be weakened as will the rest of the structure. The stone foundation, wooden structure, and iron cap are indicative of personality and confidence. Stone is representative of personal values, wood symbolizes custom creativity, and iron equates to personal strength and resilience.

I am who I am					
I am strong, built on a solid foundation.					
I am learning to accept myself.	I am experiencing a healthy relationship with my supports.	I will manage my emotions and practice healthy emotional responses.	I am experienced at tolerating and surviving crisis with the help of others.	I am good and I will be me.	
I will accept reality and who I am.		I will practice positive relationship building...		...and turn away from destructive relationships.	
I am practicing one new skill successfully.	I am learning to be realistic about my thoughts.	I am not always responsible for life's failures.	I am learning to overcome my failures.	I will think about my thoughts first not react.	I am learning new skills.
Positive regard for self: I am worthy of love	I have experienced pain and disease.	I have experienced loneliness and frustration.	I remember when I judged myself as worthless.	I am thinking about today.	I am learning to care for myself.

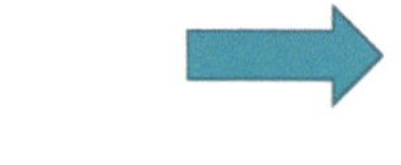

Application of Theory - Client Situation

SHELLY P., 29 year old white female, unmarried mother of two children by the same man presents to the emergency department accompanied by her parents who have requested she be admitted for mental health concerns related to drug abuse and depression. Upon assessment patient is diagnosed with substance-induced bipolar disorder. The underlying findings indicate substance abuse with crystal methamphetamine being the reported drug-of-choice used for past three years and she left all her belonging to someone she only met three months prior. She is being admitted to mental health inpatient services for further evaluation; this is her first admission to mental health services.

First session with Shelly will include an introduction to me (the therapist) and an overview of what the therapy sessions will include. The setting will be in an office with a small round table and chairs for each to sit across from one another. Face to face dialogue will take place; soft eye contact will be made with a welcoming nonthreatening smile and a handshake.

I will ask Shelly what has happened in her life that has led up to this particular meeting (patiently wait for approximately one moment). Affirmation of concern and willing to understand apprehension is expressed; and the question received a small sigh as she proceeds to share her most recent experiences involving domestic violence and drug use. I look at Shelly as asks 'how are you doing now?' Shelly offers a shallow answer stating she has nothing left to lose. I respond with I am glad you came today and I look forward to working with you helping you to overcome all of the difficulties you have experienced. Will you share with me what you believe to be a problem you would like to work through first? Her response is "I have no idea, I can't take care of my kids, I don't have a job anymore, I lost my license, I gave everything away, and I can't even get public assistance right now".

My response: thank you for sharing this, surely you

have a lot of distress; I am here to help you. Let's develop a starting point; I sense you need to be reminded of your own self worth. How do you feel about yourself right now? (Pause and listen.)

This point is where I will present the first row of the 'I am' treatment plan (diagram of solid foundation) and include a time frame that offers Shelly one hour sessions (including this one), three times a week. We will set goals today (at least one) and review the concepts to achieve together. The first goal is to obtain self regard. Homework will be provided that is simple with definitions of worth and self regard. Shelly's responsibility is to read the definition of self regard, identify and practice one point of self care before the next session. Subsequent sessions will include follow-up of her thoughts about the previous session and homework. Self disclosure may be useful to aid in the comfort Shelly needs to know she can share her darkest past and not be judged. It is important that she is able to speak of the painful experiences to discern behaviors that led up to this current life situation.

This client situation is a typical situation that involves depression, substance abuse, dysfunctional family dynamics, and lack of financial resources. Theoretically it is reasonable to build up this client's self worth, reveal maladaptive cognitions, and facilitate better choices reflecting reality. Teaching methods of acceptance through personal discovery and reflection of past events will assist client in setting and maintaining personal values. It is imperative to have a therapeutic relationship as this client has significant areas needing repair for her to become well and then begin caring for her children.

THEORY CRITIQUE

STRENGTHS OF PRACTICING this therapeutic concept are best supported by its current use today in psychiatric settings and by the evidence observed from research conducted for the three chosen theorists: Rogers's Person-centered therapy; Beck's Cognitive behavior therapy; and Linehan's Dialectical behavior therapy. Additionally, personal experience affords the orderly process of self regard; including self discovery and acceptance, current-time focusing, and self-care are effective methods of personal growth and development. Further strength is found in the educational concepts of the skill sets. Mental illness or not, these skill sets aid individuals toward realistic expectations of self and others, healthy relationships and emotions, and crisis support systems. Nursing theorist Jean Watson considers her "interpersonal and transpersonal qualities of congruence, empathy, and warmth" to Carl Rogers's views including nurses are to understand others not control them (Alligood, M. and Tomey, A., 2010). Rogers's PCT has been practiced for over seventy years strong and has been the back bone of several theorists like Watson.

Greatest limitations are commitment, time, and expense. Clearly without a commitment to this personal development plan an individual may not experience the 'actualization' of self. Time is a critical factor with weekly sessions and time spent at home with homework; essentially, the individual implements these steps into their everyday lives. As for cost, not all who will benefit from therapy have the means to pay for the needed sessions. Insurance companies including Medicare and Medicaid offer limited funds for psychotherapy. Other population limitations include illiteracy, cultural diversity, severe mental retardation, dementia, and severe psychosis.

Developing an effective and brief therapeutic process would be ideal; however, reality beckons for a lifestyle change that is not exclusive to one problem. Utilization of these theoretical concepts will be appropriate for several disorders such as: anxiety disorders, obsessive-compulsive disorders, panic disorders, posttraumatic stress disorder, chronic pain, body image, personality disorders, addiction behaviors, and mild to moderate psychosis. Groups of individuals and families will be able to practice these self-regard and personal-growth and development concepts together with the homework aspect being personalized. As the healing process begins within the participants the group dynamics will change and include regard for one another.

REFERENCES

Alligood, M. and Tomey, A. (2010). *Nursing Theorists and Their Work.* Maryland Heights: Mosby Elsevier.

Beck, J. S. (2011). *Cognitive Behavior Therapy: Basics and Beyond* (Second ed.). New York: The Guilford Press.

Boeree, C. (1998). *Carl Rogers Biography.* Retrieved from Carl Rogers: http://webspace.ship.edu/cgboer/Rogers.html

Carey, B. (2011). Expert of Mental Illness Reveals Her Own Fight. *The New York Times.* Retrieved from http://www.nytimes.com/2011/06/23/health/23lives.html?pagewanted=all&_r=0&pagewanted=print

Facuty of Department of Psychology. (2011, May 9). *Marsha M. Linehan, PhD*. Retrieved from University of Washington: https://faculty.washington.edu/linehan/Biography.pdf

Farber, B. A. (1996). *The Psychotherapy of Carl Rogers: Cases and Commentary*. New York: The Guilford Press.

History of Beck Institute. (1994). Retrieved November 22, 2014, from Beck Institute for Cognitive Behavior Therapy: http://www.beckinstitute.org/beck-institute/History-of-Beck-Institute/248/

Lineham, M. (2015). *DBT Skills Training: Handouts and Worksheets*. New York: The Guilford Press.

Prochaska, J. &. (2014). *Systems of Psychotherapy - A transtheoretical Analysis* (Eighth ed.). Stamford: Cengage Learning.